EFFECT OF ALCOHOL AND DIET ON HEALTH AND LONGEVITY

John A. Mottram

INTRODUCTION

Even if you are sceptical about my views on the relative toxicity of alcoholic drinks, you may find some thought-provoking information included here!

This booklet aims to raise your awareness of dietary hazards that we voluntarily expose ourselves to on a daily basis. You may be surprised by the book's focus on alcohol. It's a relatively overlooked cause of ill health and reduced life span. Alcoholic drinks are used as a lubricant in many social situations in the Western world. A majority of people probably give little thought to alcohol's potential to cause ill health and reduce healthy life span.

Alcohol is fairly toxic, and it's quite easy to consume amounts that negatively affect health. When digested, it is oxidized to acetaldehyde, which is about five times as toxic as alcohol itself. There are also wide variations in the sensitivity of individuals to the toxic effects of alcohol and acetaldehyde.

Many people may also be unaware that alcohol is a calorie-rich food – each gram has almost as many food calories as a gram of fat. Of course, fat in foods provides enticing taste, but is twice as calorie-rich as carbohydrate and protein. So, beware of the demon fat as well as the demon drink!

Other behavioural factors that affect health include diet and smoking. A review of these factors, and others that have an impact on healthy living, is also included.

Genetic factors must have a role shaping a person's years of healthy life. However, this booklet focuses on the main behavioural factors that are likely to affect health and life span.

Alcohol intake and smoking can both cause ill health and reduce a person's years of healthy life. Overeating is in a different category – eating is of course essential to preserve good health, but eating more than is required to maintain health can be harmful. This subject will also be discussed.

LIFE EXPECTANCY

In Western countries average life expectancies are about 75 for men and 80 for women. There are wide variations around these averages, and some life-style behaviours may well be involved. This booklet covers some possible ways to reduce lifetime-reducing risks.

I'm putting this information at the "upfront" as I believe that more people could live healthy lives until at least the age of 100 by avoiding, or severely limiting, alcohol intake and adopting some fairly simple dietary and life style changes.

You may be sceptical about some of the recommendations in this booklet. Have a look at the information I've collected and make up your own mind.

FAT IN DIET

The Food and Agriculture Organization of the United Nations (FAO) and the World Health Organization (WHO) have reported minimum requirements for fats and oils in the human diet.

According to these guidelines, for most adults dietary fat should supply at least 15 to 20 per cent of their energy intake from food.

Assuming 20% calories from fat, this means that people should obtain 80% of their calories from carbohydrate and protein. If your total food energy intake each day is 2,000 calories, then 1,600 of those food calories should therefore be obtained from carbohydrate and protein.

Minimum desirable intakes of fats and oils for infants and young children are more complex – this topic is discussed at the World Health Organization (WHO) Website.

Bear in mind that high dietary fat intake has been linked to increased risk of obesity, coronary heart disease and certain types of cancer. What constitutes excessive fat intake? In my opinion, anything over 20% to 30% of daily calories contributed by fat is too much. Among adults, there is no nutritional advantage to consuming high-fat diets, once essential energy and nutrient needs have been met.

Substantial evidence indicates that relatively high intakes of fruits and vegetables, which are sources of various antioxidants and carotenoids, reduce the risk of coronary heart disease and some cancers.

ALCOHOL

Benjamin Franklin said many years ago:

In wine there is wisdom, in beer there is freedom – but in water there is bacteria.

In his day, water supplies were often contaminated with harmful bacteria or toxic materials, so drinking wine or beer that had been treated to avoid contamination, made sense. His reasons for favoring alcohol are much less valid today, as drinking water supplies in western countries are usually safe.

Ethyl alcohol (commonly referred to as "alcohol") is the second member in the series of aliphatic alcohols. The series starts with methanol (methyl alcohol – formula CH_3OH) and proceeds through the higher members of the series by successive additions of a $>CH_2$ group.

Alcohol is usually manufactured for human consumption by the fermentation of aqueous solutions containing cane sugar (sucrose).

Alcohol-containing drinks have been in use for thousands of years. Here is a quotation from the King James Version of the English bible, originally published in 1611 AD:

A feast is made for laughter, and wine maketh merry: but money answereth all things.

Note that ethanol is not a carcinogen, but the first metabolic product of ethanol during digestion is acetaldehyde, which is toxic, mutagenic and carcinogenic.

Here are the definitions for these terms:

Toxic – of or relating to or caused by a toxin or poison. A toxin is a chemical compound that when ingested can cause injury or death.

Mutagenic – A mutagen is a physical or chemical agent that changes the genetic material of an organism and thus increases the frequency of mutations, and causes cells in the body to be damaged.

Carcinogenic – A carcinogen causes, or tends to cause, cancer.

IS ALCOHOL GOOD FOR HEALTH?

There is a widespread belief that alcoholic drinks, particularly wine, can have a positive effect on health. This is contrary to research showing that alcohol has negative effects on health at any intake. In other words, NONE is better!

An agency of the World Health Organization (WHO) has recommended the following limits for low risk drinking of alcoholic beverages by humans:

Men: no more than two drinks a day

Women: No more than one drink a day

Over 60's: No more than one drink a day

A Google search on the Internet will find many references on alcohol consumption limits.

A sceptic could argue that "no more than one drink a day" may mean "no alcoholic drinks at all per day." My argument is, if alcohol has known toxic effects, why consume any? This is my recommendation – what each person does is up to him or her. But, please be aware of the potential risk to health and longevity of regular alcohol consumption.

The WHO agency defines a standard drink as follows:

One 12 ounce serving of beer (5% alcohol)

One 5-ounce glass of wine (12% alcohol)

1.5 ounces of 80-proof liquor (40% alcohol)

DEATHS CAUSED BY ALCOHOL

The organization Alcohol Concern has reported that alcohol-related deaths in the UK exceed 30,000 a year.

On the World Wide Web, Medscape has reported that in 2001, alcohol use was responsible for about 75,000 preventable deaths in the USA.

Worldwide, the number of deaths attributed to alcohol is estimated to be about a million a year.

The head of Emergency Services at Royal Sussex County Hospital (UK) has said: "I cannot underestimate the importance of alcohol in the workload of emergency departments – we would be out of business if it was not for alcohol."

EXERCISE AND HEALTH

How important is exercise? There is some doubt on its value, in spite of the current popularity of regular vigorous exercise.

Physical exercise of some sort is probably important to maintain good health. Most people enjoy exercising, be it on the golf course, in the gym or by walking or jogging. A key question is: how much exercise is necessary to maintain good health? Some people may exercise to burn off the excess calories consumed by eating and drinking too much. A sensible, but possibly boring, alternative would be to consume just enough food calories to maintain a healthy weight throughout life.

In his book "The Exercise Myth" published in 1984, cardiologist Dr Henry Solomon threw doubt on the idea that vigorous exercise is necessary to maintain the heart in good health. He suggested that regular energetic exercise in a gym, or running, would not necessarily prevent the eventual onset of heart disease. He recommended limited physical exercise, such as walking, but thought that even the risks incurred by people who were sluggish "couch potatoes" were minimal.

Here is what he says in a summary:

THIS IS NOT AN ANTI-EXERCISE BOOK

It is simply the other side of the exercise story, the side few people have heard and some don't want to know. There is no mystery to exercise. You don't have to be initiated into membership, to believe in esoteric claims, or practice arcane rituals. Whatever benefits the human body derives are yours whenever you take a good brisk walk or enjoy yourself – without pushing yourself – at some other sport you enjoy.

The facts don't obviate the pleasure of exercise, but they do say exercise is dangerous when it's done for the wrong reasons. The truth can protect you from the claims and aims of others, and perhaps from yourself. You can exercise for fitness and for pleasure, and you can do it safely.

Dr. Solomon wrote that the consensus of experts is that there is little or no evidence that exercise training increases the coronary collateral circulation in humans.

My studies indicate that other factors are more important for health and longevity. As mentioned earlier, these are: avoidance of alcohol and other relatively toxic materials.

Since Dr. Solomon's book was published, the possible dangers of inactivity causing blood clots forming in the legs have been discovered. This is more likely to occur during long flights. Information on this topic is available on the Internet at the American Society of Haematology website.

The following table shows data on average healthy weights for men and women:

AVERAGE HEALTHY BODY WEIGHTS

Height Inches	Men Pounds	Women Pounds	Difference Pounds
58		115	
60		120	
62	137	125	-12
64	142	133	-9
66	148	140	-8
68	154	146	-8
70	160	153	`-7
72	167	159	-8
74	175		

The above average values were copied from the WHO website. Note that the reference also includes data for "small" and "large" frame humans. I chose "average frame" values.

BODY MASS INDEX (BMI)

It is well established that body weight can have an effect on health and longevity. The BMI is an easy way to figure whether your weight is in a healthy range. It is calculated from your weight and height as follows:

Metric Units – Divide body weight in kilograms by the square of height in metres. The formula is:

BMI (Metric Units) = W / (H * H)

US Units – Divide your weight in pounds by the square of your height in inches, and divide the result by 703. The formula is:

BMI (US Units) = (W / (H * H)) / 703

If these formulas seem confusing, there are many BMI calculators available on the Internet which will do the calculation after you input your weight and height. After working out your BMI, you can see where it fits into the following table.

The United States Centre for Disease Control has published these BMI ranges:

BMI Range	Category
18.5 – 24.5	Normal
25.0 – 29.9	Overweight
30.0 – 38.9	Obese
40 and above	Extreme obesity

The data above are valid for both males and females, including children. Some sources show different BMI ranges for males and females, and for children under 20. However, the above values are adequate for general guidance in most cases.

How reliable is BMI as an indicator of body fatness?

The correlation between the BMI number and body fatness is fairly strong; however the correlation varies by sex, race, and age. These variations include the following examples:

- At the same BMI, women tend to have more body fat than men.

- At the same BMI, older people, on average, tend to have more body fat than younger adults.

- Highly trained athletes may have a high BMI because of increased muscularity rather than increased body fatness.

It is also important to remember that BMI is only one factor related to risk for disease. For assessing someone's likelihood of developing overweight or obesity related diseases, the US National Heart, Lung, and Blood Institute guidelines recommend looking at two other predictors:

- The individual's waist circumference (because abdominal fat is a predictor of risk for obesity-related diseases).

- Other risk factors the individual has for diseases and conditions associated with obesity (for example, high blood pressure or physical inactivity).

What are the health consequences of overweight and obesity for adults?

Overweight and obese individuals are at increased risk for many diseases and health conditions, including the following:

- Hypertension

- High LDL cholesterol, low HDL cholesterol, or high levels of triglycerides)

- Type 2 diabetes

- Coronary heart disease

- Stroke

- Gallbladder disease

- Osteoarthritis

- Sleep apnea and respiratory problems

- Some cancers (endometrial, breast, and colon)

AIM FOR A HEALTHY BMI

When you eat more food than your body needs in its daily activities, the excess is accumulated as body fat. Of course, regular exercise will burn up calories, but it's probably more important to watch what you eat. In my opinion, it is pointless to consume more calories than the body needs, and then try to burn off the excess by exercising, or worse – consuming some heavily advertised elixir that promises you can lose weight while eating all you want!

If your BMI is within the normal range, you're likely to be achieving the right balance between food input and your body's energy needs. When your BMI is above average, the excess food energy is converted into added body weight.

WHAT TO DO WHEN YOUR BMI IS HIGH

Perhaps you may decide not to change anything, but it would be sensible to understand how you got there, and how to reduce your BMI to achieve a healthy weight. Remember – excess weight can lead to heart disease and reduced life expectancy.

The food choices we make can affect weight gain, because equal quantities of fat and alcohol provide about twice the calories that carbohydrates and protein do. This is shown in the following table:

One gram of:	Calorie Contribution:
Fat	9
Carbohydrate	4
Protein	4
Alcohol	7

MORE INFORMATION ON BMI

As mentioned earlier, fats and alcohol pack about twice the calories as carbohydrates and protein.
How high fat content snacks can contribute to calorie intake is shown in the table below, compared to non-fatty snacks.

All figures below are for four-ounce portions:

	Grams of fat	Calories
Roasted peanuts	56	884
Milk chocolate	37	537
Apple, orange or carrot	< 0.3	< 54

This table illustrates a common truth – fatty snacks can add significantly to your calorie intake, while fruit and vegetables are low in calories and fat. One high-fat snack can supply 20 to 40% of your daily calorie requirement. Note also that a single glass of wine or a can of beer contribute 100 to 150 calories.

CARNIVORES, HERBIVORES & OMNIVORES

These are all mammals, classified by their principal sources of food.

Carnivores, such as tigers, kill and eat other animals. They have teeth designed for catching and killing live prey, and dismembering their bodies. Their large intestines are short in relation to their body size, probably to avoid the development of toxic chemicals from their protein-only diet.

Herbivores such as cows, eat grass, and have multi-compartment stomachs for breaking down and digesting their high-fibre foods.

Humans are classed as omnivores – their diets can comprise foods from both animal and vegetable sources. Their digestive systems have a relatively long small intestine that is required to break down largely vegetable foods. This suggests that an optimum diet for humans should be largely based on vegetables and fruit, with limited amounts of protein.

TOBACCO

Research data clearly show that smoking shortens the life expectancy of most users. People who wish to live a long and active life should avoid tobacco altogether. The extent to which the smoking habit reduces health in later life, and life expectancy, varies depending on many lifestyle factors, including alcohol intake.

The dangers of using tobacco products are so well known that they will not be discussed further. Much information is available on the Internet for those who are interested.

AFTERTHOUGHTS

Finding a way to live a long and healthy life is a work in progress. Some pointers on significant lifestyle issues have been covered in this booklet.

There is a widespread belief that about 8 hours sleep a day is needed to maintain the body in good health. Most of us know people who sleep only 4 to 6 hours most nights. Whether they will live long lives is unknown. No doubt future research will unravel this. For the time being I'll accept the belief that my brain needs 6 to 8 hours sleep to keep me healthy.

It has become common in recent years to see people sucking on bottles of water. This is presumably based on the belief that toxins can be flushed out via the kidneys. The kidneys will not flush out fat-soluble toxins, which may finish up being stored in the liver. In my opinion, the value of excess water intake is uncertain.

MORE INFORMATION

An excellent review of the negative impact of alcohol, and other factors, on health is at www.cancerwa.asn.au. When at the web site, select "Reduce Your Risk" and select from a menu of risk factors.

A vast amount of information on health issues is available on the Internet. Use a Google search to explore health topics you're interested in.

"The Exercise Myth" by Dr. Henry Solomon, referred to in the text, is a cardiologist's sceptical view on the need for energetic exercise.

Almost daily, the news media report on a multitude of nostrums and quick fixes that are claimed to reduce the risk of cancers, heart attacks and ills of all sorts. There are also frequent descriptions of how to quickly (and effortlessly!) reduce weight. Be sceptical of these reports, and explore their validity on the Internet.